The National Primary Care Research and Development Centre is a Department of Health-funded initiative, based at the University of Manchester. The NPCRDC is a multi-disciplinary centre which aims to promote high-quality and cost-effective primary care by delivering high-quality research, disseminating research findings and promoting service development based upon sound evidence. The Centre has staff based at three collaborating sites: The National Centre at the University of Manchester, The Public Health Research and Resource Centre at the University of Salford and the Centre for Health Economics at the University of York.

For further information about the Centre or a copy of our research prospectus please contact

Maria Cairney
Communications Officer, NPCRDC
The University of Manchester
5th Floor, Williamson Building
Oxford Road
Manchester M13 9PL

Tel: 0161 275 7633/7601

Contents

About the authors

Robert Boyd is a Principal of St George's Hospital Medical School. Until recently he was Chairman of the Management Board of the NPCRDC.

Tom Butler is Senior Fellow for Development and Dissemination at the NPCRDC.

Linda Gask is Senior Lecturer in Psychiatry and a Joint Appointment between the NPCRDC and the University Department of Psychiatry.

Caroline Glendinning is Senior Research Fellow at the NPCRDC.

Jennie Popay is Associate Director at the NPCRDC and Professor of Community Health Studies at the University of Salford.

Anne Rogers is Senior Research Fellow at the NPCRDC and Reader in Sociology at the University of Salford.

Martin Roland is Director of Research and Development at the NPCRDC at the University of Manchester and Professor of General Practice at the University of Manchester.

Bonnie Sibbald is Senior Research Fellow at the NPCRDC and Reader in Health Services Research at the University of Manchester.

David Wilkin is Chief Executive of the NPCRDC and Professor of Health Services Research at the University of Manchester.

1

Introduction and overview

Tom Butler

This briefing paper is the second of a series that is intended to provide policy makers, commissioners, managers, primary care professionals and user organizations with up-to-date briefing on important issues for primary care development. The aim is to discuss policy issues and their implications at national and local levels and to review published research that may inform future decision making.

Primary care is increasingly centre stage in NHS plans for the future of health care in the UK. The Department of Health has set out plans for the long-term development of the NHS by four key policies: The Health of the Nation, Caring for People, The Patient's Charter and a primary care-led NHS. The NHS Executive published a framework of future planning that sets out the medium-term priorities for services.[1] These are: a primary care-led NHS; mental health; effectiveness; patient and public empowerment; continuing care and human resources. This was followed by a consultative paper published by the NHS Executive (1996) in a response to a consultative process established by the Secretary of State for Health.[2] This paper set out a framework for an emerging agenda on primary care which highlighted seven key themes. These were: resources, partnership in care, developing professional knowledge, patient and carer information and involvement, securing the workforce and premises, better organization and local flexibility.

Primary care is not only a key health policy commitment for the NHS but it is also a priority for service planning for the future. However, these ideas are painted with a broad brush and leave many health professionals speculating about the form and content of future services. For those with responsibility for commissioning and purchasing services, as well as those who deliver services to patients, there is a vacuum in understanding what a primary care-led NHS means for them and those who rely on their services. A recent DoH publication prepares the way for new legislation without structural reorganization.[3]

The purpose of this briefing paper is twofold. First, to explore seven aspects of the move towards a primary care-led NHS and second, to contribute to the debate including an assessment of the future role of the National Centre in informing future discussions with research evidence. This collection of papers draws on a range of research perspectives from within the National Primary Care Research and Development Centre to explore and clarify some of the concepts and implications of this major policy initiative by the NHS Executive.

In the first paper Martin Roland and David Wilkin examine the rationale for moving towards a primary care-led NHS and consider the aims of the NHS, the special features of primary care and the future relationship between the two. They argue that while it is likely that an increased focus on primary care will improve care, this is not guaranteed. The slogan of a 'primary care-led NHS' needs to be backed by evidence to ensure a beneficial outcome.

Anne Rogers and Jennie Popay consider user involvement in primary care in the second paper in this collection. The paper describes three distinct ways in which users have or could become involved in primary care services. The first two approaches are associated with past or current practices and the third approach is a response to rapid change and innovation in health care. Rogers and Popay argue that for a primary care-led NHS to produce real patient benefits, a change in professional–lay relationships is needed.

The third paper in the collection is by Robert Boyd, who looks at the challenges posed by the move towards a primary care-led NHS from the perspective of a hospital-based paediatrician. He argues that a primary care-led NHS will be judged by four criteria: the effects it produces on accessibility and acceptability of services, quality of care provided and cost-effectiveness. Boyd sounds a warning note against being too self-congratulatory. He argues that as primary care leadership develops, its ability to correct NHS failures must be enhanced and demonstrated.

Bonnie Sibbald considers key issues in the move towards a primary care-led NHS with regard to innovation and experimentation with the disciplinary mix and roles of the general practice teams. In considering the future direction of primary care development, Sibbald highlights the need to develop an evidence base to underpin skill mix change.

Mental health presentations to primary care is well understood in the literature. The paper by Linda Gask argues that we know relatively little about the patients' views of the mental health services they receive from primary care. She examines the changing role for two groups of patients: those with mild and moderately severe problems and those with severe, complex and enduring mental health problems. Gask argues that primary care has a key role to play in ensuring that historic divisions between professional disciplines, rigid diagnostic decisions or arbitrary age barriers do not serve patients well. By contrast Gask proposes a new view of the service provision with an emphasis on innovation and co-ordination.

Some of the same themes are explored by Caroline Glendinning in her analysis of the changing interface between primary care and social care. She looks at the boundaries between health and social care and argues that changes at these boundaries are likely to present some of the main challenges to primary care over the next decade. Glendinning identifies a number of factors that will shape the relationship between health and social care, including demographic trends, cost containment and the changing balance between public and private responsibilities. Within this policy context she examines the consequences for service users and the implications for primary care overall, including the impact of changing residential services, the growth of the mixed economy of provision, formal and informal health and social care.

The final paper in this collection is by Martin Roland. It argues the case for a research perspective on the changing face of primary health care and the relationship to secondary and social care. Roland sets out the role of the National Primary Care Research and Development Centre as an NHS-funded independent research agency, working to inform the debates and plans on primary care health policy and professional decision making, through the use of evidence rather than rhetoric. The Centre has five main programme areas and is currently conducting 25 research projects related to primary care.

The move towards a primary care-led NHS presents many opportunities for improved services for patients through local innovation and demonstrations of good practice. Equally it runs the risk of being introduced in an atmosphere of rhetoric and hyperbole that reinforces the well-recognized gap between research and practice in health care decision making. The National Primary Care Research and Development Centre has an important role to play to support and drive research and development initiatives in primary care. This collection of papers is a contribution to help health professionals to close the gap between research and practice in order to take a more informed part in the debate on the move towards a primary care-led NHS.

REFERENCES

1 NHS Executive. (1996) *Priorities and Planning Guidance for the NHS: 1997/99.* HMSO, London.

2 NHS Executive. (1996) *Primary Care: The Future.* HMSO, London.

3 Department of Health. (1996) *Choice and Opportunities.* HMSO, London.

2

Rationale for moving towards a primary care-led NHS

Martin Roland and David Wilkin

Primary care provides first-contact, generalist continuing care to the great majority of health problems presented to the NHS. Since 1948, a key function of primary care has been to act as a gate-keeper to specialist services. Primary care is, in general, located geographically close to patients' homes. It treats people in the context of their communities, and is potentially more accountable to its local community.

The UK model of primary care is widely admired in other countries, and in many there is a move to increase the primary care orientation of their health care systems (e.g. the United States, and the countries of Eastern Europe).

It is now proposed that the focus of health care in the UK should move further towards primary care – through changing the focus of both provision and purchasing of health care. If primary care is 'good', will more of it be 'better'? In this paper, three questions will be considered in discussing the rationale for moving towards a primary care-led NHS:

1   What are the aims of the health service?
2   What are the special features of primary care?

3   How can the aims of the health service be more closely approached by increasing those features which relate to primary care?

The paper acknowledges the general practice-based team as the foundation of primary care in the UK, but also recognizes the increasing diversity of community-based providers, and also the diversity of potential purchasing arrangements within the NHS.

WHAT ARE THE AIMS OF THE HEALTH SERVICE?

The NHS should provide care which has the following characteristics:

- equitable access to all population groups
- acceptable to the population
- responsive to the needs of the population
- cost-effective
- accountable.

In moving towards a primary care-led NHS, these are features which should be the subject of analysis. A successful primary care-led NHS should increase these characteristics of health care in the UK.

WHAT ARE THE SPECIAL FEATURES OF PRIMARY CARE?

There are a number of features of care which are particularly described as characterizing primary care. Although these are not necessarily unique to primary care, they are the features which primary care practitioners believe characterize their disciplines.

The first key feature of primary care is easy access. Because primary care services are locally based, patients' ability to access care is improved when compared to services provided at a greater distance.

The second key feature of primary care relates to the fact that care is provided by generalists rather than specialists. The specialist has a narrow range of problem-specific skills. The generalist in contrast has a broad range of competencies, suited to dealing with both well-defined and undifferentiated problems. Particular features of care provided by generalists[1,2] are that it:

- emphasizes the whole person, and the context in which that person lives
- is person centred as opposed to disease centred
- provides a comprehensive range of services
- provides care over a long period (sometimes called longitudinality)
- provides continuity of care
- coordinates the care for individual patients.

In the rest of this paper, the extent to which the key aims of the health service might better be achieved by increasing *primary care* will be discussed. In the discussion, the distinct purchaser and provider functions of primary care need to be separated.

HOW WILL THE HEALTH SERVICE IMPROVE BY BECOMING MORE PRIMARY CARE FOCUSED?

Will equity improve?

One of the outstanding features of the NHS is that it provides care to almost the entire population through registration with the general practitioner (GP). Registration provides access to both primary care and secondary care. This is in marked contrast to some countries, for example the United States, where significant parts of the population have very poor access to health care.

In terms of access to primary care, there are a number of significant threats to equity if the purchasing and providing roles of primary care practitioners increase. First, it is essential that the NHS is able to recruit a high-quality workforce to all parts of the country. Current recruitment problems within general practice, combined with progressive retirement of overseas doctors who have tended to practise in urban areas, means that it may become difficult to staff deprived and inner city areas. If the focus of provision of care within the NHS shifts towards primary care, then equity of access may reduce in areas where it is difficult to recruit a high-quality primary care workforce. The problem of inner cities may be further compounded by changes in the hospital sector. To some extent, the variable quality of inner city general practice may in the past have been counterbalanced by the presence of high-quality teaching hospitals in large conurbations. The reduction in number and size of these large institutions may be occurring precisely in the locations where general practice is least able to adapt and change.

The second risk to equity of access to primary care lies in further developments in GP fundholding. There is a risk that GP purchasers will 'cream skim' when faced with significant budgetary pressure, i.e. discourage registration of expensive patients. This has not been a problem in the UK to date, but is a substantial problem in the United States. Mechanisms need to be developed to avoid this.

Will access to secondary care be influenced by moves towards a primary care-led NHS? Fundholding has led to some inequities, in that patients of fundholding practices have had improved access to certain types of secondary care services. However, fundholding has been patchy, and if GP involvement in purchasing becomes more evenly spread in a primary care-led NHS, then equity may improve. Some inequities may be inevitable in a market-driven system: indeed, some would argue that it is the very presence of inequity which acts as a driver for overall improvement.

Will care become more acceptable to the population?

The public has, in general, substantial confidence in GP services. However, there is a growing demand for specialist services, reflected in rising rates of referral to hospital. This is due in part to the growing awareness by the public of high-technology care from which they could benefit. While patients appreciate the provision of local services, they have less access to specialists in this country than in most other developed countries, and it is not clear that provision of an increasing amount of care in the community will be acceptable to patients. They will need to be confident that primary care is not second-class care.

Will care become more responsive to local needs?

There is no reason to believe that secondary care is organized to be responsive to local needs. Often primary care is not either. However, an increased focus on primary care practitioners as both purchasers and providers of health care could increase responsiveness to local needs. Increasing the primary care focus of the NHS implies moving closer to the needs and views of patients, though current mechanisms for listening to the needs of patients are poorly developed. The assumption that a primary care-led NHS is automatically closer to a patient-led NHS may not be translated into reality without specific incentives being introduced for primary care staff to become more responsive to their communities.

General practitioners need not become more involved in needs assessment. In many cases, this is better carried out in collaboration with public health physicians. However, a focus on primary care will increase the opportunities for identified local needs to be addressed, through changes to primary care services, or through primary care-led purchasing of secondary care. These gains are unlikely to be realized unless there is greater involvement of and accountability to local communities.

Will care become more cost-effective?

In considering this key question, the purchaser and provider functions of primary care need to be considered separately.

Does primary care-led purchasing lead to more cost-effective purchasing? This is a key question in relation to fundholding. The answer for individual patients is probably 'Yes'. By and large, GP fundholders have shown themselves to be successful entrepreneurs in securing improved services for their patients. What is less clear is how good GPs are as purchasers for whole populations – e.g. are they more likely to neglect certain groups than health authorities? In addition, it is not clear whether GPs will remain efficient purchasers under conditions of budgetary restraint. On the whole, GP fundholders have been under less financial pressure than health authorities since 1991. Funding pressures are now becoming more evenly distributed, and it is not clear whether small size will then prove to be an advantage or a disadvantage. However, as secondary care becomes more specialized, the primary care values of continuity, coordination and provision of comprehensive care are certainly ones which are increasingly needed. The increase in available, effective (but costly) secondary care procedures argues strongly for a generalist coordinating the care of individual patients.

Will primary care-focused provision improve the cost-effectiveness of delivery of care within the NHS as a whole? The international evidence suggests that it will: primary care-focused health care systems are certainly cheaper to run, and are probably (though with some exceptions) more cost-effective than specialist-oriented systems. However, we already have a health care system which is more primary care focused than that in almost any other developed country. It is not clear whether the argument can be extrapolated further still – with increasing cost-effectiveness as more and more care is transferred to the primary sector. Some argue that much care provided in the primary sector is ineffective,[3] and that to increase the volume of this care will not improve the overall cost-effectiveness of the NHS.

The answer to cost-effective delivery of primary care will depend on resource transfer and targeting. If care is progressively transferred to an already stretched primary care sector, then quality may decline, and care may become less cost-effective. This question needs to be looked at critically for each service. In some areas, e.g. follow-up of patients with some chronic diseases, there may well be opportunities to provide more cost-effective care than that currently provided by specialists. However, it is important if resources are shifted to reflect changes to the location of care, that they are shifted so far as possible into services which are at least as likely to be effective as those previously provided in secondary care.

Will care become more accountable?

At present, the performance of primary care is less closely monitored than that provided in secondary care. If this does not change, then transfer of care to the primary sector is likely to result in a loss of accountability. However, an increasing focus on the purchasing of specific services from primary care (to a specification) will increase the accountability of primary care.

Accountability should be to the population being served, though in practice it is often to managers acting essentially on behalf of the community. However, it is known that NHS managers may not always have the same priorities as NHS patients.[4] Therefore, if mechanisms are introduced to increase the accountability of primary care as the focus of care shifts to that sector, there are real questions about who primary care is to be accountable to. There are no inherent reasons why a primary care focus should not lead to greater accountability to local populations than that currently provided in secondary care. In some respects, the small size of primary care organizations may make accountability easier to achieve.

CONCLUSION

There are strong reasons for believing that an increasing primary care focus could improve care within the NHS. However, transfer of the focus of purchasing or providing to primary care will not guarantee improvements in equity, acceptability, responsiveness, cost-effectiveness or accountability. In each case, careful consideration needs to be given to how an increasing primary care focus will improve care. In this age of evidence-based care, the political slogan of a 'primary care-led NHS' needs to be backed by evidence to ensure a beneficial outcome.

REFERENCES

1 Royal College of General Practitioners. (1995) The Nature of General Medical Practice. Report from General Practice, No. 27. RCGP, London.

2 Starfield B. (1992) *Primary Care: Concept, Evaluation and Policy.* Oxford University Press, Oxford.

3 Maynard A, Bloor K. (1995) Primary care and health care reform: the need to reflect before reforming. *Heath Policy.* **31**: 171–81.

4 Smith CH, Armstrong D. (1989) Comparison of criteria derived by government and patients for evaluating general practitioner services. *BMJ.* **299**: 265–70.

FURTHER READING

Gordon P, Hadley J. (1996) *Extending Primary Care: Polyclinics, Resource Centres, Hospital at Home.* Radcliffe Medical Press, Oxford.

Meads G (ed). (1996) *Future Options for General Practice.* Radcliffe Medical Press, Oxford.

3

User involvement in primary care

Anne Rogers and Jennie Popay

The last decade has witnessed a growth in the involvement of users in all areas of the health service, including primary care. Such involvement has been most pronounced in relation to maternity, mental health and disability services. In the primary care sector the inclusion of users has been less marked. This may partly be a result of the pattern of the utilization of primary health care services, which are used intermittently and infrequently by some groups of people. For this reason it has sometimes been assumed that the extent to which users can become involved in primary care is limited.

The move towards a primary care-led NHS is seen by many as moving towards a patient-led NHS. Primary care practitioners are regarded as more responsive to the broad needs of their individual patients and local communities, and the importance of their role has been highlighted by GPs' increasing role in purchasing.

In this paper, we describe three distinct ways in which users have or could become involved in primary care services. The first two are approaches which characterize past and current service delivery. The third approach, by extending the participation of lay people in primary health care, has the potential to meet the demands of a rapidly changing and innovative health care sector. We argue that, for a primary care-led NHS to produce real patient benefits, a change in the professional–lay relationship is needed to allow real participation of patients in their health care.

PATIENT COMPLIANCE AND 'HOLISM': A PROFESSIONALLY DEFINED AGENDA

A traditionally accepted view among some GPs has been that ascertaining the views of patients is important for ensuring compliance with medical treatment and advice. Understanding what triggers a consultation has clear utility for patient management. The GP or other primary care workers may more appropriately intervene in a patient's efforts to cope with illness if she or he has the knowledge and awareness of the patient's view of health and illness, and their expectations and reasons for seeking help. More recently there has been some adoption of 'holism', a philosophy which takes cognizance of the patient's environment, spiritual and emotional needs through multi-disciplinary team working. These approaches have been viewed as a means of overcoming some of the shortcomings of a purely bio-medical model.[1]

Both of these developments have brought with them a greater sensitivity to patient-centred working. They include a refound interest in the Balint model, stress the importance of uncovering the 'undiseased' private aspects of patients' lives and are informed by a commitment to listening and 'learning from the patient'. The value and rationale for including a lay perspective in primary care has changed with changes in health policy. An underlying ethos of understanding patients in order to ensure compliance with medication or as a result of new disciplinary philosophies has more recently been augmented with concern for ascertaining consumer views as a measure of the quality of services.

THE IMPACT OF CONSUMERISM

A different approach to user involvement from that described above has followed in the wake of the 1990 and 1991 NHS reforms, changes in the commissioning and delivery of services and the presence of a broader consumerist philosophy. This is evident in the Patient's Charter:

> *We will be encouraging health authorities to continue and expand their use of questionnaires and surveys to find out what you think of the current services and to get your suggestions of how things could be better done.*

The terms and conditions of the 1990 GP contract appear to have had a positive impact on consumer perceptions of the quality of care that they receive, with improved satisfaction levels in relation to waiting and consultation times.[2] More generally, patient satisfaction has come to be seen as an attribute of the quality of the service and as a legitimate health care goal in its own right. This has meant increased involvement of patients in determining aspects of the delivery of care. A number of practices and a plethora of evaluation research have sought to include patients' views of services in order to implement changes and reshape services. There have for example been changes in the organization of antenatal, maternity and infant care. In one practice this has taken the form of the reorganization of antenatal bookings and classes and an undertaking to respond quickly to infant illness.[3] Interpersonal and communicative skills on the part of the practitioner have been found to be of particular value to patients, as are conveniently situated and accessible services.[4]

LIMITATIONS OF THE PROFESSIONAL AND CONSUMERIST APPROACHES TO USER INVOLVEMENT

Despite undeniable advantages, there are nonetheless limitations to the utility of both of these models of user involvement in primary care, which as they stand do not adequately challenge the range of barriers in the way of the optimal use of services or maximize the potential of citizen participation in primary health care:

> *Whilst patients' evaluations have been an important aspect of contemporary general practice and are a significant aspect of modern service delivery, there is some concern that patients' beliefs and evaluations may not be embodied in crude expressions of satisfaction collected via structured surveys. We do not currently know how patients evaluate 'care' and whether current popular evaluation tools accurately embody the motives, intentions and beliefs of service users.*[5]

Whilst policy changes have introduced structural reforms the practical constraints of choice in the primary care market have not been addressed, and there is evidence to suggest that the public do not make market-style choices when selecting their general practitioner.[6] Moreover, opportunities for participation are frequently restricted to exercising the option of 'voting with one's feet' or 'exit/choice' as a result of major dissatisfaction with the service in a system where choice is restricted.[7]

PATIENTS AS EXPERTS AND PARTNERS IN PROVIDING PRIMARY CARE

Both the professional and consumerist approaches have tended to prioritize the issues which providers or policy makers have viewed as important about the delivery and organization of services. To an extent, user, provider and commissioning perspectives may well coincide. (The growth in primary care counselling is an example here.) But there is potentially more to a primary care agenda which seeks to maximize user participation and roles in providing for care.

Firstly, there is scope for an extension of the consumerist perspective, in defining quality standards and pursing effectiveness. Questions about the value of medical care and procedures have rarely been seen as suitable topics to follow up with users.[8] Yet appropriateness and acceptability of medical interventions to patients are at the heart of patient care.[9] Patients can contribute to efforts being made to promote the practice of evidence-based medicine.* If dissemination of the effectiveness, advantages and disadvantages of clinical interventions relevant to primary care were made more widely available, patients would be in a better position to evaluate the evidence for or against health care options. This would assist them to become more equal partners with primary care workers in taking health care treatment and management decisions.

Secondly, policy makers are concerned with managing the demand for services effectively and meeting unmet need. At the levels of professional practice and research and development, an understanding from the patient's perspective of the relationship between health problems, the experience of ill health, and the use of primary care is important to both commissioners and providers of health care in devising more appropriate services and sensitive resource allocation. Such an understanding would allow for services to be better orientated to the way in which people actually use them.†

* There is evidence to suggest that this may decrease demand, as indicated by the use of an experimental video about the treatment of benign prostate problems.

† For example, in the area of lay knowledge about mental health there has been some suggestion that those seeking help for psychological problems may be seeking out tangible support (e.g. access to material and social resources) rather than directly provided therapeutic support.[10,11] A more in-depth understanding of how women understand, make decisions about and experience pregnancy has also been important in reorienting the provision of maternity and antenatal support within primary care.

Thirdly, the inclusion of lay knowledge has the potential to act as a complement to medical and professional knowledge in a primary care health care system which aspires to lead the NHS. This requires more than the ascertaining of the views of patients about existing services. Lay people, like professionals, are providers as well as recipients of care. They have experience of self-care and care for others and are regularly involved in providing advice about and taking responsibility for health and illness. An in-depth understanding of the nature of lay knowledge and active involvement is needed to inform the design and delivery of services. The challenge for primary care is the extent to which it is able to nurture and maximize such input in a way which ensures lay people's full participation in the management of their care alongside professional primary health care workers.

We have as yet little knowledge of the rights and obligations which users of primary care sense they have, and what they perceive their role to be, or indeed in what ways and to what extent people wish to participate in primary care. It has been suggested that collective community participation at the organizational level of primary care has been inhibited because of a bio-medical perspective and an individualistic focus within practices. A failure to involve key groups more fully might in part be a function of a clash between 'paternalism and participation'.

If we are to maximize patients' involvement in an NHS which becomes more focused on primary care and the communities which those primary care teams serve, then future efforts need to address more fruitfully the way in which we might involve users as equal partners and participants, alongside health care professionals and policy makers, in their own care. Those efforts need to be targeted most at those who feel disenfranchised or have been marginalized from mainstream services (e.g. black and minority ethnic groups) and those in greatest health need.

REFERENCES

1 Royal College of General Practitioners. (1995) The Nature of General Medical Practice. Report from General Practice, No. 27. RCGP, London.

2 Williams B. (1994) Patient satisfaction: a valid concept? *Soc. Sci. Med.* **38**(4): 509–16.

3 Mellor J, Chambers N. (1995) Addressing the patient's agenda in the reorganisation of antenatal and infant health care: experience in one general practice. *Br. J. Gen. Pract.* **46**: 423–5.

4 Lewis J. (1994) Patients' views on quality care in general practice. *Soc. Sci. Med.* **39**(5): 655–71.

5 Williams S, Calnan M. (1991) Key determinants of consumer satisfaction with general practice. *Fam. Pract.* **8**: 237–42.

6 Leavey R, Wilkin D, Metcalfe D. (1989) Consumerism in general practice. *BMJ.* **298**: 737–9.

7 Brown I. (1994) Community and participation for general practice: perceptions of general practice and community nurses. *Soc. Sci. Med.* **39**(3): 335–45.

8 Wensing M, Grol R, Smits A. (1994) Quality judgements by patients on general practice care: a literature analysis. *Soc. Sci. Med.* **38**: 45–53.

9 Calnan M. (1988) Towards a conceptual framework of lay evaluation of health care. *Soc. Sci. Med.* **27**: 927–33.

10 Pilgrim D, Rogers A. (1993) Mental health service users' views of medical practitioners. *J. Interprofessional Care.* **7**: 167–76.

11 Rogers A, Pilgrim D. (1996) Understanding and promoting mental health: a study of familial views. *HEA Family Health Research Reports.*

4

Challenges to a primary care-led NHS: a medical specialist's view

Robert Boyd

The criteria by which a primary care-led NHS should be judged include its effect on accessibility and acceptability of services, quality of care and cost-effectiveness. In this paper the moves towards a primary care-led NHS will be considered under these headings, taking the perspective of a hospital paediatrician with a major interest in primary care health services research.

ACCESSIBILITY AND ACCEPTABILITY OF SERVICES

Does a non-hospital site confer automatic benefit? There is a widespread belief, well supported by anecdotal historical experience, that services delivered in primary care are more patient sensitive. However, the belief that hospitals are so institutionalized that they cannot improve is probably wrong (e.g. hospital-based palliative care teams, breast screening, open-access paediatric units, hospital-based primary care). This view may lead to unwise service development – e.g. provision of 'hospital' services on a non-hospital site for philosophical rather than access reasons.

The increase in the size of primary teams which will inevitably follow a primary care-led NHS may also diminish the historically greater patient responsiveness within primary care. This needs to be addressed directly through charter standards, market testing of services in relation to patient responsiveness, and monitoring by CHCs and others. In the hospital specialist's view a community-related specialist service may be better provided by a specialist team or facility headquartered in a hospital unit rather than by a fresh primary care development, the primary care focus being ensured by purchasers. Furthermore, imaging and other equipment-based diagnostic facilities of increasing importance will be cheaper if located where usage can be maximized, usually in a hospital.

Is a primary care-based service 'best'? Acceptability of primary care provision depends on a balance between the two contradictory trends: geographical accessibility versus perceived quality. Patients want prompt, friendly, accessible care, preferably at home or close to home. They also want to know they have had the 'best' care before accepting inevitability. The rise of litigation, of specialty-related support groups for patients, of media consideration of patient biographies, and of patient-accessible IT will increase the conflict. Primary care will need to be able to advise patients wanting super-specialist care and will increasingly find that patients do not accept a 'no' to referral.

QUALITY OF CARE

'Technical' or clinical quality has been given less attention in considering quality indicators for primary care than in secondary care. It also risks being undervalued in purchasing decisions made by primary care. The following specific challenges to quality may follow from a move towards primary care purchasing.

Maintenance of specialty expertise

This is the sum of expertise available in primary, secondary and tertiary care, for the management of patients falling into a particular specialty area. A real risk here is of 'de-professionalization'. The key driver for quality of the workforce within a specialty area especially, but not exclusively, medical, is the sense of belonging to a professional subgroup. A doctor working in any specialty sees him or herself primarily as a paediatrician, urologist or oncologist. It is also important to remember that much expertise of nurses and therapists flows from their membership of specialist services.

This self-identification and classification into specialties is bolstered by formal processes, e.g. specialist registration and training programmes and by the existence of royal colleges and specialty societies. It is reinforced by the personal relationships which follow from shared training experiences, from patronage of various kinds and from joint attendance at conferences, committees and meetings. It is strengthened by the titles and contents of journals that specialists read, and also by academic departmental structures and networks, both national and international. Specialty expertise is used by management at all levels to develop policy, and especially to troubleshoot.

The real challenge is how to maintain the quality which grows out of the peer group concept while making the specialties more responsive to the priorities of addressable need as perceived from primary care.

At the national level, this requires a two-way process. Specialty groups, in conjunction with generalists, need to address the epidemiology of need relating to their specialty. They need to be set the 'exam question': what elements of your expertise could be better delivered, directly or indirectly, in primary care? What are the constraints which need to be tackled in achieving it? A primary care-led NHS will lose credibility if specialty perceptions of poor 'technical' quality of specialty-related provision in primary care

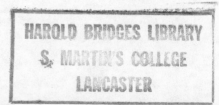

are not listened to, quantified and addressed (e.g. can age-generic primary care demonstrate that it provides good-quality paediatric care – most national systems do not believe so).

At local level, audit systems, guidelines and purchasing plans need to be tested by how well they operate for a given specialty area across sectors in an illness episode or chronic care mode. Outreach clinic value should be maximized by timetabled specialist/GP interaction so that the secondary care team understands better the primary care perspective and its technical problems and vice versa. There is good evidence that this is not happening at present. Furthermore, outreach clinics must provide the technical backup which specialists need in order to be able to provide an effective service.

Maintaining the capacity for specialty-driven service innovation

Many (perhaps most non-generic) primary care innovations have in the past been driven by the specialties (although, critically, with input from pioneers within primary care), e.g. asthma guidelines (British Thoracic Society), quality management of diabetes (British Diabetic Association), encouragement of breast-feeding (paediatrics), safe childbirth (obstetrics), paramedics (A&E consultants). In the author's view, the biggest single challenge to a primary care-led NHS is how to maintain, focus and enhance the peer group specialty-driven enthusiasm for service improvement.

Maintaining a knowledge-based workforce

Within a specialty, consultants retain and improve their quality predominantly through peer interactions. There may be a major cultural difference between primary and secondary care in this regard. Questioning of GPs suggests that informal consultation between partners in the presence of a specific patient is surprisingly uncommon. In hospital, discussing individual patients with

colleagues is commonplace. These unscheduled learning interactions are at risk if consultants have more commitments outwith
their units in primary care. A diminution of the learning ethos
within a specialty unit damages the workforce quality of all health
professionals working in that area. However, learning should be a
two-way process. Encouraging positive early career experiences is
important and vigorous efforts should be made to expand junior
medical staff rotations between hospital and general practice.

COST-EFFECTIVENESS

Will a primary care-led NHS be cheaper? The majority of current
NHS costs is staff pay and of this, within the service as a whole,
the bulk is expenditure on nursing. A service in which most care
is delivered in primary care may increase global (i.e. financial and
non-financial use of resources by all parties) costs. This is partly
because the carer to dependent ratio is unlikely to fall when patients
are distributed over many habitations rather than in a Nightingale
ward, an effect which has been particularly evident in the deinsti-
tutionalization of psychiatric care. However, in addition, care costs
will fall on a much wider range of individuals and institutions,
especially on family networks and on social care organizations. The
removal of double infrastructure costs for patients resident at home
rather than in hospital may lead to some real saving. However, pro-
tection against violence for health care professionals may be more
expensive and more difficult to achieve in a primary care setting.

Some assume that a primary care-led service would invest less in
the marginal returns of poorly treatable illness (excess intensive care
for the very tiny neonate, or the irreversibly damaged, some can-
cers, advanced cardiovascular disease, etc.). Again, there are con-
flicting trends but at present increasing demand for marginal care
(e.g. equal access for over 70s) appears likely to dominate. The
fact that the GP rather than the hospital or health authority will
make decisions on the use of resources will not self-evidently

increase or reduce demand for expensive care of only marginal benefit to the patient.

There is also a risk that purchasing from primary care may over-develop provision for conditions which bear heavily on primary care because of their frequency (backache, minor depression) even when evidence of effectiveness (physiotherapy, counselling) is slight and the need to purchase care for rare, more severe, problems is underestimated (e.g. psychosis). This effect may also blunt the rapidity of response to new medical challenges (e.g. from the unusual infections which are likely to increase with globalization of movement and with less diverse food chains) or opportunities.

THE BROADER VIEW

Many devotees of the NHS claim that our health care system is a world leader and that primary care is the jewel in its crown. A cooler look is less flattering. Japan has an equally cheap system but one that is more 'effective' as judged by the overall, if 'unfair', test of life expectancy. Consumer satisfaction may be greater in most of our EU partners but care is more expensive. In specific specialties, our outcomes may be worse than those of many other OECD countries, e.g. cancer treatment results. Our health inequalities may be widening.

As primary care leadership in the NHS develops, its ability to correct NHS failures must be enhanced and demonstrated:

* together with HAs, primary care purchasers must ensure the continued development of high-quality secondary care. Specialty peer groups will need to be enhanced and refocused, not weakened, to achieve this
* primary care must engage more vigorously in the purchase of the public health agenda (like secondary care, primary care is therapy, not prevention, minded)

- monitoring of the care delivered by primary care needs to be much more effective, while not damaging the individual patient responsiveness that is primary care at its best – a difficult task.

5

Skill mix and professional roles in primary care

Bonnie Sibbald

The move towards a primary care-led NHS implies an expansion in the numbers and types of staff working within primary care, and the development of new professional roles. The key drivers behind these changes are:

- rising demand and cost of care, which has increased interest in the possible economies to be made by shifting care from expensive to cheaper health professionals
- NHS policy changes which encourage a shift from hospital-based to community-based care, thereby increasing the volume and range of services demanded of primary health care teams
- a fall in medical manpower in general practice, consequent on a recent decline in recruitment to the specialty and a shift towards part-time working related to the increasing proportion of female doctors. A fall in medical manpower can be sustained without loss in service provision only if care is shifted from doctors to nurses and allied health professionals.

The impetus for change has been facilitated by:

- growth in GP fundholding, which makes it easier for GPs to purchase the staff and services they need to diversify and expand their care provision
- GP-led purchasing of community and secondary health care services, which makes it easier for GPs to shape the ways in which these services are provided. For example, GPs have been enabled to bring community-based and secondary care professionals into the practice to provide services.

This paper outlines key issues which need to be considered as the move towards a primary care-led NHS increases innovation and experimentation with the disciplinary mix and roles of general practice teams.

AN EVIDENCE BASE FOR SKILL MIX CHANGES

Ideally the size and composition of the primary care team should be governed by research-based evidence of how skills may best be distributed among health professionals in order to optimize the cost-effectiveness of health service delivery. In practice most, if not all, the major changes in skill mix within primary care have not been adequately evaluated. Examples include the substitution of nurse practitioners for general practitioners, the widespread use of practice-employed counsellors to treat minor mental illness, and the delegation of traditional health visitor roles to less highly qualified community nurses, auxiliary nurses and nursery assistants.

Recent years have seen a belated upsurge of research into skill mix, but this research is largely discipline specific – focused on the role of an individual discipline (e.g. general practitioner) and its boundaries with other disciplines (e.g. nursing). Little attention has yet been given to the impact of collected changes in skill mix on primary care services as a whole. It remains unclear whether task delegation/substitution or specialization within primary care teams are cost-effective strategies.

Costs are easier to measure than the quality or cost-effectiveness of services. Health service managers under pressure to make year on year efficiency gains are sometimes compelled to alter staff skill mix in the absence of objective evidence of how this may affect the quality or cost-effectiveness of service provision. This fuels the belief of many health professionals that reforms are driven more by the need to save money than by consideration for the overall quality of services. Loss of morale and a deepening resistance to change are a natural consequence of disbelief in the rationale for change.

CHANGES IN ROLES: THE NEED FOR A CLEAR VISION

Although changes in skill mix have not been guided by research-based evidence of their cost-effectiveness, neither have they been guided by a coherent vision of the future role of primary care. Insufficient attention has been given to the impact of ongoing and proposed NHS reforms on the professional values and capacity for change of primary health care staff.

General practitioners

As highly qualified *generalists*, GPs are able to deal with the most common health problems in the population. They are the only primary health care professionals qualified to make a full initial assessment of patients' health needs. As *gatekeepers* to secondary health care, GPs coordinate service delivery and ensure expensive specialist services are used appropriately. Although the cost-effectiveness of gatekeeping has not been fully assessed, international comparisons suggest a powerful effect. The quality and cost-effectiveness of health service provision may therefore suffer if nurses, specialists and professionals allied to medicine (e.g. counsellors) substitute for GPs in providing first-contact care.

A second area of concern is the tension experienced by many GPs in acting both as purchasers and providers. GPs have traditionally been person-centred physicians, motivated to achieve the greatest possible health gain for each individual patient. The move to make GPs responsible for resource allocation within the practice (through budget setting) and outside the practice (through the commissioning of community and secondary care services) is perceived to run contrary to the ideal of person-centred care. GPs find it difficult to reconcile the often competing demands of maximizing both the health of individual patients and the health of the patient population as a whole. Many believe that economic models cannot be embraced within the doctor–patient relationship without irreparable harm to the latter. This is important, not only in terms of enlisting GP support for NHS reforms, but because the quality of the doctor–patient relationship is among the most important factors determining patient satisfaction and confidence with health services.

Primary health care nurses

GP fundholding and GP-influenced purchasing of community nursing services has generally encouraged a breakdown in the boundaries between health visitors, district nurses and practice nurses to achieve greater flexibility in the deployment of nurse skills. GPs have contracted to bring health visitors into the practice to manage their health promotion services and to remove the boundaries between district nurses and practice nurses, encouraging the former to undertake delegated medical tasks within the practice and the latter to provide nursing care in the home. Nurses increasingly undertake medical tasks delegated by the doctors and work under the day-to-day clinical direction of doctors rather than nurses. In essence, nurses are encouraged to become medical assistants.

If, as some suppose, nursing and medicine are conceptualized as the performance of tasks, then nurse–doctor substitution would be relatively unproblematic. However, nursing and medicine have distinctive values and cultures which shape care provision. There is real concern that policies which encourage nurses to become medical assistants will erode nursing autonomy and values, so impoverishing the quality of patient care. However, it is also plausible that nurse–doctor substitution may enable nurses to achieve greater autonomy and bring their values to bear on a wider range of health services. The question is whether nursing values will shape, or be shaped by, current trends in task delegation and substitution.

General practice managers

The management of general practice services has undergone rapid change in response to the NHS reforms of the 1990s. The transformation of FPCs to FHSAs and the merger of FHSAs with DHAs have demanded that managers move from administration to operational management and from operational to strategic management. General practices similarly have needed to develop skills in operational and strategic management in order to respond effectively to NHS contract changes and the demands of an internal market. The GP contract of 1990, the introduction of fundholding, and the planned introduction of total purchasing all serve to give practice managers greater power to determine the size and composition of primary care teams. But are practices equipped with the skills needed to identify and manage desired changes in skill mix?

Management capacity has lagged behind organizational change, particularly within general practice. Managers who have 'grown up' with the health service have generally lacked opportunities to develop their skills in operational and strategic management. Managers imported from outside the health service have generally lacked training in how to apply business management principles to general medical services. The management of change in skill mix demands high-quality managerial skills which are, as yet, under-developed in many general practices.

FUTURE DIRECTION

The further development of a primary care-led NHS demands:

- a solid evidence base to underpin skill mix change. Major changes in professional roles should not be initiated without good evidence of cost-effectiveness. Health professionals need to be persuaded that proposed changes can enhance health outcomes for patients, or at least not diminish the quality of patient care
- respect for the professional values of service providers. Future primary care organizations need to acknowledge and accommodate the difficulty experienced by many primary health care professionals in reconciling person-centred care with population-centred care. Nursing and medicine have distinctive cultures and should not be viewed as interchangeable
- improved management skills in general practice. There needs to be greater investment in developing the operational and strategic management skills of practice managers if they are to respond effectively to the demands of the internal market and primary care-led NHS
- widespread changes in skill mix which additionally have major implications for:

    - manpower planning (need for forward planning in recruitment and training policies to meet the demand imposed by altered skill mix requirements in primary health care)
    - in-service training (need to (re)train existing professionals wishing to extend or alter their roles in primary health care provision)

– professionalization/accreditation (need to agree standards
for the accreditation of newly emergent professional groups
[e.g. counsellors] and existing professionals who want to
undertake radically new roles [e.g. nurse practitioners]).

FURTHER READING

GMSC. (1996) Medical Workforce Task Group Report, February 1996. British
Medical Association, London.

Huntington J. (1995) *Managing the Practice: Whose Business?* Radcliffe Medical
Press, Oxford.

Richardson G, Maynard A. (1995) Fewer Doctors? More Nurses? Discussion
paper No. 135, Centre for Health Economics, University of York.

Royal College of General Practitioners. (1995) The Nature of General Medical
Practice. Report from General Practice, No. 27. RCGP, London.

Starfield B. (1992) *Primary Care: Concept, Evaluation and Policy.* Oxford University Press, Oxford.

6

Mental health perspectives on a primary care-led NHS

Linda Gask

Over the last 30 years a great deal of epidemiological work has been carried out into mental health problems in primary care. We know, for example, that more than 90% of mental 'illness' is treated by GPs, yet the vast bulk of resources earmarked for mental health care are still tied up in the hospital in-patient services. We also know a great deal about how GPs respond to people who present to them with mental health problems and the ways in which the system responds to these problems along the 'pathway' to secondary care, first described by Goldberg and Huxley.[1]

Changes in policy and service provision have resulted in people receiving care from primary care, secondary care, social care, and voluntary and self-help organizations, and achieving lifetime patterns of care which differ considerably from those of the past. Primary care is now rightly seen as having a more important role than traditional psychiatric services in coordinating care and maintaining long-term support for people with all types and severities of mental health problem.

In an increasingly primary care-led NHS, are primary practitioners prepared and equipped to extend this role, both in terms of providing care for people with mental health problems, and in taking an extended role in purchasing mental health care? The interest of GPs in the mental health problems of their patients remains very variable, for reasons that are still unclear.[2] Attempts to improve the mental health skills and knowledge of GPs are taking place but have a considerable way to go and 'top-down' initiatives are probably ineffective.[3] There is also still a great deal that we do not know about what happens to patients along the way. For example, we know that patients in touch with psychiatric services prefer the care that they get from their GP.[4] However, we still know very little about what the patients themselves think about the mental health care that they receive solely within primary care. It is too complacent to think that because people continue to visit the doctor it means they are happy with what they are offered. Perhaps they feel that they have no real choice, or they do not know what the options are. 'Traditional' methods of assessing patient satisfaction using questionnaires are also fundamentally flawed because they are developed from the professional view of what good care is.[5] The growth of GP fundholding, and more recently the developments in total purchasing of mental health services, have recognized the lack of needs assessment at a local level within primary care, but have often still to address the involvement of patients in decision making. The recent OPCS surveys of psychiatric morbidity in Great Britain will assist in service planning by providing predictions of population-based morbidity, but cannot be a substitute for local knowledge and patient insights.[6]

The drive towards evidence-based practice has also highlighted that within the mental health field much of the research into effectiveness of treatment and outcome has not actually been carried out within primary care. Drug trials have been largely conducted with highly selective and atypical secondary care populations. This must lead to the conclusion that much of the received wisdom about, for example, treatment of depression in primary care with 'adequate' doses of antidepressants,[7] is not as firmly based in experimental research as it might be.

Definitions of mental illness and mental health are controversial but the author proposes to discuss in turn the changing role of primary care for people with more severe and enduring mental health problems followed by those with problems of mild to moderate severity. It is crucial to recognize first of all that 'severity' cannot be defined by diagnosis but must also take into consideration issues of potential risk to the person and to others, duration and pattern of illness, the burden to carers and the response of the system itself.

PRIMARY CARE AND PEOPLE WITH SEVERE AND ENDURING MENTAL HEALTH PROBLEMS

People with severe and enduring problems are usually (but certainly far from always) in touch with both primary and secondary care. We need to foster schemes that encourage close links between primary care, secondary care, voluntary agencies and social services to assist in the development of locally comprehensive networks of care for this group. 'Shared care' schemes, where GP, CPN and psychiatrist liaise closely, are promising developments, although practice-based case registers (for example of schizophrenia) have some ethical implications which have yet to be addressed. Where such systems are developing, research is needed to determine why some systems of care seem to work well and others fail so badly. Coordination of care with secondary care and the voluntary sector is very patchy, and better coordination is a key benefit which should follow from an NHS which becomes more strongly oriented towards primary care.

PRIMARY CARE AND PEOPLE WITH MILD AND MODERATELY SEVERE MENTAL HEALTH PROBLEMS

Many people with apparently mild or moderately severe mental health problems may nevertheless require more specialized help at some point in their 'illness career'. Unfortunately, the skills required are not always possessed by local psychiatrists and clinical psychologists remain in short supply. Could primary care have a key role in negotiating for the provision of evidence-based therapeutic skills at a local level? Often what is available locally, for example for the patient with unremitting depression, is no better than the GP has already tried, and the growth of inaccessible specialist tertiary referral centres, which may not necessarily offer cost-effective or evidence-based care (rather like traditional alcohol treatment units), must be resisted.

Primary care has a key role to play in ensuring that historical divisions, whether based on professional distrust (psychiatrists and psychologists), inappropriately rigid diagnostic decisions (general psychiatric and substance misuse services) or arbitrary age cut-off (child and adult services, old-age psychiatry), do not continue to allow people to slip through the net or receive services that do not address their needs.

MENTAL HEALTH PROMOTION

Many people working within primary care teams may have great enthusiasm for and some expertise within the field of mental health promotion and prevention of anxiety or depression.[8] Nevertheless, the evidence for the effectiveness of such interventions remains limited at the present time,[9] and must be weighed cautiously when planning how to provide truly comprehensive care for people with mental health problems.

PRIMARY CARE AND PEOPLE WITH COMPLEX MEDICAL AND SOCIAL NEEDS

Another challenge lies in the need to address the complex needs of people with a mixture of physical, social and mental health problems. A broader view of what is meant by 'mental health' within the primary care team could lead to improved acknowledgement of and better coordinated mental health care for the large number of people with emotional difficulties seen not just by doctors but also by health visitors, practice nurses, midwives, district nurses and school nurses. Most of this 'morbidity' falls within the remit of 'anxiety' or 'depression' but the simplicity of the diagnostic terminology tends to diminish the complexity of the problems faced (bereavement, terminal care, support to carers and families, family problems) and promotes over-dependence on medical models of assessment and treatment.

The 'facilitator', who aims to identify and meet practitioners' training needs, appears a promising way to develop mental health skills within primary care.[10] However, recognition is needed that workers themselves need continuing support and supervision if they are to employ these skills effectively. Some practices employ their practice counsellor to fulfil this role, while others turn to clinical psychologists, community psychiatric nurses or psychiatrists, whichever locally can offer the interest and appropriate skills. Primary care-led purchasing offers real opportunities to coordinate care, not only within the health services, but also to develop local links with social services, voluntary and self-help sectors, to share the burden of care effectively. Local planning arrangements for social services may not always make this an easy task.

NEW INITIATIVES IN MENTAL HEALTH PURCHASING

New initiatives in extending 'traditional' fundholding and developing total purchasing and local commissioning provide the biggest opportunity for changing the face of primary mental health care. These are not, however, without their own potential threats. GPs cannot ignore that good mental health care requires a 'spectrum' of facilities including, when necessary, in-patient beds.[11] It could be potentially disastrous for the community if resources were diverted to counselling services (not yet evidence based) away from in-patient care without first ensuring that other services (e.g. assertive outreach care for the severely mentally ill – which is evidence based) are first in place.

It is going to be a major challenge to ensure that a primary care-led NHS can communicate well enough within itself to avoid wasting money and time on re-inventing the wheel and making the same mistakes over again. If this does not happen, we risk a fragmented system of care, riven with inequalities, where those with more severe problems or a greater need will not be prioritized. Research and development initiatives must recognize and address this problem before it is too late. This means that evaluation must both keep pace with and respond to the needs of the changing agenda in mental health care.

REFERENCES

1   Goldbert D, Huxley P. (1992) *Common Mental Disorders: A Bio-Social Model.* Routledge, London.

2   Kendrick T, Sibbald B, Burns T *et al.* (1993) Role of general practitioners in the care of long-term mentally ill patients. *BMJ.* **302**: 508–10.

3   Turton P, Tylee A, Kerry S. (1995) Mental health training needs in general practice. *Primary Care Psychiatry.* **3**: 197–200.

4   Pilgrim D, Rogers A. (1993) Mental health service users' views of medical practitioners. *J. Interprofessional Care.* 7: 167–76.

5   Williams B. (1994) Patient satisfaction: a valid concept? *Soc. Sci. Med.* **38**: 509–16.

6   OPCS. (1995) *Surveys of Psychiatric Morbidity in Great Britain.* Bulletin No. 1. The prevalence of psychiatric morbidity among adults aged 16–64 living in private households in Great Britain. HMSO, London.

7   Paykel E, Priest R. (1992) Recognition and management of depression in general practice: consensus statement. *BMJ.* **305**: 1198–202.

8   Murray R (1995) *Prevention of Anxiety and Depression in Vulnerable Groups.* Gaskell, London.

9   Canadian Task Force on the Periodic Health Examination. (1995) *The Canadian Guide to Clinical Preventive Health Care.* CCG-P, Ottawa.

10   Armstrong E. (1995) *Mental Health Issues in Primary Care: A Practical Guide.* MacMillan, London.

11   Department of Health. (1996) *The Spectrum of Care: Local Services for People with Mental Health Problems.*

7

The changing interface between primary care and social care

Caroline Glendinning

INTRODUCTION

This paper examines the boundaries between primary health services and social care. It identifies the factors currently affecting these boundaries and discusses the implications for primary care services and patients. Changes at this boundary are likely to present some of the main challenges to primary care over the next decade, and will be crucial in considering how a primary care-led NHS can lead to improved care across the whole of health and social care.

A number of major demographic and policy developments are likely to affect the boundaries between primary health and social care services in the future.

Demographic trends

Demographic changes are likely to place considerable pressures on both the funding and the organizational capacity of statutory health and social care services. The numbers of people aged 85+ will increase fivefold between 1961 and 2026;[1] for at least some of these future generations of older people, prolonged periods of insecurity, unemployment and deprivation during their working lives may result in greatly increased needs for health and other services in advanced old age. The age profile of ethnic minority communities is likely to change particularly rapidly; the development and coordination of services to meet the needs of an ethnically diverse older population will become an increasing priority.

Cost containment

There is growing convergence within OECD countries towards a view that the political limits to further expansion of public expenditure have been reached, and that welfare states should increasingly play enabling and empowering, rather than direct service provider, roles. Future changes of government are likely to see only a change of emphasis, rather than a direct challenge, to these assumptions.

The drive to contain costs has two consequences. First, it creates pressure to define more clearly and tightly the boundaries around the responsibilities of specific services so as to ensure that money is not 'wasted' by performing tasks which should be provided by another organization. Secondly, it places greater emphasis on the 'gatekeeping' activities of primary and community health service practitioners who assess needs and decide whether access to more expensive services is appropriate. These pressures are likely to fragment rather than improve the coordination of services for individual users.

Redrawn boundaries between public and private responsibilities

Across all OECD countries there is interest in finding new ways of combining public with private provision. This includes both the introduction of private funding into health and social care services, through mechanisms such as private insurance, co-payments and charges for services; and the redesignation of certain types of treatment or care as private and personal, rather than public, responsibilities (non-clinical care for older people is a topical example of this).

CHANGING BOUNDARIES BETWEEN PRIMARY CARE, SECONDARY CARE AND SOCIAL CARE

Within the NHS, the boundaries between primary and secondary health services are widely regarded as important in the delivery of effective and efficient health services. However, these boundaries are far from static. The transfer to primary and community health sectors of services hitherto carried out in hospital settings are already making these boundaries much more fluid. Developments associated with a primary care-led NHS are likely to have a continuing impact on the boundaries between primary and secondary health services, and should, if adequately resourced, increase opportunities to provide high-quality care outside hospital settings.

Many of these changes also have implications for the provision of social care. Changes within the acute hospital sector (earlier discharge, the development of 'hospital at home' schemes and the attrition of long-stay in-patient provision, for example) not only have major implications for primary and community health services but also create additional needs for formal and informal social care.

In contrast to the fluid boundaries between primary and secondary health services, the pressures to maintain clear distinctions between health needs and social care needs are substantial. The different funding mechanisms and organizational structures which govern the NHS and local authority services create pressures to define what is not health care, or what is not social care. Demands for services which exceed the capacity of health or social services authorities to meet them thus create 'perverse incentives' to place responsibility for particular services or types of care in someone else's organization and on someone else's budget. For example, responsibility for providing assistance with personal care, especially bathing, has long been contested between health and social services organizations. Similarly, the development of guidelines on eligibility for continuing NHS care[2] is a response to the tendency of many health services purchasers over the past decade to define high levels of long-term dependency as 'social' rather than 'health' needs, regardless of the actual nursing or clinical intervention which may be required.[3]

THE CONSEQUENCES FOR SERVICE USERS

Older frail or disabled people and those involved in providing help and support on an informal basis do not distinguish between health care needs and services and social care needs and services. However, the pressure to define and strengthen the boundaries between health and social services are likely to work against other stated service objectives, such as creating a 'seamless' service, achieving 'continuity of care', or developing 'user-led' services. Three aspects of this problem can be identified.

First, the distinction between health and social care has become increasingly problematic for service users because of the widespread introduction of charges for local authority domiciliary, respite and day care services.[4,5] Thus help with bathing will be free of charge if it is regarded as a 'health' need and provided by community nursing services, but is likely to incur charges if it is a 'social' need met by the local authority home care service or day centre. This major difference in the conditions of access to similar services provided by the NHS and local authorities raises important questions of equity; is likely to affect user choice and demand for services; and constrains opportunities for skill mix and substitutions across organizational boundaries.

Secondly, the distinction between health and social care services complicates enormously the process of finding out about services and how to obtain them. Over the past two decades, studies of disabled children,[6,7,8] disabled adult,[9] frail older people[10] and informal carers[11] have repeatedly reported difficulties in finding out what services are available, in what circumstances and through what means of access.

Thirdly, fragmentation between health and social care services increases the number of different agencies and professionals who need to be told about sometimes very personal circumstances and needs. It also creates major problems of coordination in the delivery of services. In addition, it is likely to affect the acceptability of services if, for example, frail or vulnerable people are faced with a series of different people (home care worker, community nurse, bathing assistant, night sitter, emergency alarm call warden) all coming into their homes on a regular basis.

THE IMPLICATIONS FOR PRIMARY CARE

The trends described above have a number of implications for primary health care services.

The role of residential services in meeting long-term care needs

Despite the rhetoric of 'community' care, meeting convalescent, respite and long-term health care needs increasingly involves residential and nursing home provision as well as domiciliary and community-based services. GP fundholders and total purchasers

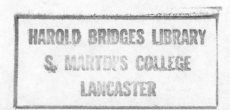

have particular responsibilities for the purchase of long-term, respite and convalescent services in residential and nursing home settings – a responsibility which until the early 1980s lay with health authorities and which since 1993 has rested largely with local authority social services departments. Primary care purchasers will therefore need to ensure that the principles which informed the 1993 'community care' changes – those of choice, user involvement, needs-led assessment and service packages and clear quality assurance mechanisms – equally govern the residential care services which they purchase or commission.

Furthermore, as the providers of primary health care to people living in non-hospital settings, GPs may increasingly find themselves acting as advocates for older people for whom hospital discharge is imminent. This role will be particularly important if eligibility for continuing NHS care is in dispute, in order to ensure that very frail and vulnerable people are not the subject of undignified boundary disputes between health and social care providers.

'Mixed economies' and internal markets

Through the introduction of care management, the 1993 'community care' changes emphasized the importance of integrating a variety of different services, from different service providers, to meet the particular needs of individual people. This was part of the explicit encouragement of a 'mixed economy' of social care providers. In contrast to the NHS 'internal market', social services departments have been encouraged to purchase services in an 'external' market of independent commercial and not-for-profit providers.

Providers of social care services therefore include not only local authority social services departments, but also increasingly include voluntary and private commercial organizations, self-help and advocacy organizations. If primary and community health service providers and purchasers are to negotiate the interface with formal social care services, they will therefore need to engage with these other commercial and not-for-profit social care providers.

Formal and informal health and social care

The bulk of social care (most recently estimated to have an annual value of £33.9–£39.1 billion) is provided on an informal, unpaid basis, by spouses, children and parents.[12] The 1993 community care changes have placed even greater reliance on informal carers.

With a growing proportion of the population needing long-term personal care and support, the pressures which have already led social services departments to transfer responsibility for social care to informal carers are increasingly likely to be felt by primary and community health service providers as well. These pressures are likely to be particularly acute in the areas of personal care and low-technology nursing and medical interventions. Primary care professionals will need to give priority to improving the practical and moral support they can give to informal and family carers in these new tasks. This pressure is likely to be increased by the implementation in April 1996 of the Carer's Act, which has at last entitled carers to an independent assessment of their own needs.

CONCLUSION

One dimension of this overarching policy involves locating decisions about treatment and care as close as possible to individual patients. This involves increasing the role of primary health service providers, through GP fundholding and other commissioning activities, in shaping secondary health services and community health services. This creates tremendous challenges and opportunities for primary care practitioners. As providers, they are likely to be increasingly influenced by boundary disputes beyond their control. There is therefore an urgent need to explore what role primary care might play, through purchasing, commissioning and provider activities, in improving the coordination and coherence of health and social care services.

REFERENCES

1   Grundy E. (1995) Demographic influences on the future of family care. In: Allen I, Perkins E (eds), *The Future of Family Care for Older People*. HMSO, London.

2   Department of Health. (1995) *NHS Responsibilities for Meeting Continuing Health Care Needs*. HSG(95)8. DoH, London.

3   Darton R, Wright K. (1994) Changes in the provision of long-stay care, 1970-1990. *Health and Social Care in the Community*. 1(1): 11–26.

4   NCC. (1995) *Charging Consumers for Social Services*. National Consumer Council, London.

5   Chetwynd M, Ritchie J, in collaboration with Reith L, Howard M. (1996) *The Cost of Care*. JRF and Policy Press, Bristol.

6   Glendinning C. (1983) *Unshared Care*. RKP, London.

7   Glendinning C. (1985) *A Single Door: Social Work with the Families of Disabled Children*. Allen and Unwin, Hemel Hempstead.

8   Beresford B. (1995) *Expert Opinions*. JRF and Policy Press, Bristol.

9   Parker G. (1993) *With this Body: Caring and Disability in Marriage*. Open University Press, Buckingham.

10 Baldock J, Ungerson C. (1994) *Becoming Consumers of Community Care*. JRF, York.

11 Twigg J, Atkin K. (1994) *Carers Perceived*. Open University Press, Buckingham.

12 British Medical Association. (1995) *Taking Care of Carers*. BMA, London.

8

Evidence-based policy development: the role of the National Primary Care Research and Development Centre

Martin Roland

Research over the past twenty years has consistently shown great variations in the patterns of delivery of care. These variations have been found in all countries, in primary care, in secondary care, and, as seen in the variation in hospital referral patterns, at the interface between primary and secondary care. Demonstration of these wide variations in medical practice has convinced policy makers that health services can be made to operate more efficiently. A key part of the UK government's policy to improve health care in this country is to shift the balance of care to the primary sector.

One cannot conclude from past research that the balance between secondary and primary care in the UK is right in one direction or the other. Examples can be found of both over- and under-provision of specialist care within the NHS at present. Governments in many parts of the world have become convinced that health services may become more cost-effective by shifting the balance from secondary to primary care. Among Western industrialized countries, the UK already lies at one end of a spectrum, with our population having relatively less access to specialists' care than people in most other countries. It may well be possible to improve the overall cost-effectiveness of care by shifting the balance further from secondary to primary sectors. However, it would be unwise to assume that care can be moved from one sector to the other without any loss in quality. In making such decisions, the focus must be on the ability of each sector to provide cost-effective care, and research has a key role in inform-ing policy in this area.

There are within the UK a number of powerful drivers promoting the move of care from the secondary to the primary sector. First, there is the clearly formulated government policy to give primary care greater responsibility in leading the direction of care in the NHS. This relates both to the provision of care within the primary sector itself, and to the expanding roles which GPs are being given in purchasing secondary care.

Second, there are changes in professional practice. In part, these relate to technical advances which have and continue to reduce the requirement for hospitalization for many procedures, e.g. laparo-scopic surgery. However, they also relate to technological changes within primary care, e.g. the development of patient testing, the development of information technology, and the improvement of primary–secondary care IT links, including telemedicine.

Third, there are changes in public expectations, with an expec-tation that treatment, where possible, should be provided near the patient's home. Provision of a wide range of services is increasingly seen as one of the markers of quality in general practices.

The forces which are tending to move care from the secondary to the primary sector – government, professional, fiscal and con-sumer led – are likely to stay. However, if care is to move from secondary to primary sectors and quality be maintained, it is likely that resources will need to move as well. It seems unlikely that there is sufficient slack within primary care for quality to be maintained unless shifts of care from the secondary sector are accompanied by an appropriate transfer of resources. Research is needed to identify where those resources would best be placed.

Research, development and dissemination at the National Primary Care Research and Development Centre aims to contribute to the formulation of evidence-based policy in these areas. There are five major programmes of work at the National Centre:

1 Population health and demand for care
2 Commissioning, provider organizations and service delivery
3 Workforce and professional roles
4 Quality in primary care
5 Interfaces between primary care, secondary care and social care.

In each of these areas, we will carry out new research relevant to the needs of the NHS. We will disseminate the findings of our research, and the work of others, to as wide an audience as possible. We also aim to be involved in promoting significant innovative examples of knowledge-based service development. Through each of these, we hope to contribute with others to the future development of the NHS, with its strong focus on primary care, which we believe can continue to act as a model for the developed world.

Index